Building a Fitness Empire with Social Media

Table of Contents

Social media is not just an activity; it is an investment of valuable time and resources. Surround yourself with people who not just support you and stay with you, but inform your thinking about ways to WOW your online presence

— Sean Gardner

Chapter 1. Introduction

Presenting to you an exciting Special Report that shines a light on the intertwined worlds of fitness and digital tech - "Building a Fitness Empire with Social Media". This is not just for fitness enthusiasts but for anyone who has ever been drawn to the idea of marrying health and the digital space. Get ready to embark on a fascinating journey of how the health and wellness industry is leveraging the power of social media to create thriving business empires. Here, we'll delve into electrifying case studies, ground-breaking strategies, practical tips and tricks, and insightful interviews with industry pioneers. By the time you're done with this Special Report, you'll feel like you're halfway through creating your very own empire! Immerse yourself in the world where fitness meets the digital revolution, and be prepared to be inspired and empowered. You don't want to miss out on this invaluable guide that could spark your next big idea!

Chapter 2. The Power of Social Media in Today's Fitness World

In an age where consumers are increasingly turning to the digital realm for all of their needs, it is prudent to point out how social media is redefining traditional boundaries when it comes to fitness. From nurturing communities of like-minded individuals to offering quick workout fixes and nutrition tips at the tip of one's fingertips, social media has truly revolutionized the way we perceive and interact with the concept of health and wellness today.

2.1. The Emergence of Social Media in the Fitness Industry

Social media platforms began to steadily influence various aspects of our lives in the late 2000s. The fitness industry, in particular, discovered a goldmine when it recognized the potential of these platforms to attract a global audience. The ability to create and share highly visual content resonated with aspirational fitness enthusiasts who were eager to embrace digital solutions for their health and wellness journeys.

The most significant pivot came with the rise of smartphones, which enabled users to access these social media platforms from the comfort of their homes or offices. It brought a high degree of convenience, allowing users to consume fitness-related content whenever they wished. Health advisors, trainers, and fitness influencers could now connect with millions of people worldwide, offering tips, advice, and motivation.

2.2. The Shift in Consumer Dynamics

What was once a private, individual endeavor, fitness soon turned into an interconnected, social activity, inspiring friendly competitiveness and camaraderie. The Instagram-fueled craze for an "Instagram-worthy body" or simply sharing your fitness progress became more than just a passing trend. It started a dialog, an exchange of ideas, and a source of motivation.

Individuals were no longer just passive consumers of content but active participants. They started sharing their own progress, fitness routines, successes, and even failures, transforming fitness into a more relatable and achievable concept. This reciprocal interaction established a symbiotic relationship between the influencers and their followers, fostering a sense of community.

2.3. Identifying the Power of Social Media

One cannot underestimate the power of social media when it comes to its effect on the fitness domain. It has successfully managed to:

1. Reach a global audience: This is crucial for the fitness industry, where the target market is not confined to one geographic area. The wide networking capabilities of social media have helped fitness experts, influencers, and brands connect with potential customers around the globe.

2. Influence and inspire healthy behaviors: Internet-based interventions have become effective in promoting physical activity. Regular posts, live sessions, online challenges are some of the ways in which social media encourages users to make healthier lifestyle choices.

3. Generate revenue: For fitness businesses, social media provides an avenue for advertising and brand promotion. From selling workout plans and e-books to merchandise and fitness equipment, social media platforms ensure a steady income stream.

This power of social-media-fitness symbiosis has triggered the rise of many innovative branded content, social media marketing agencies, and fitness applications, significantly contributing to the economy and marking an era of millennial culture.

2.4. Conclusion

The fitness world continually evolves, and social media has been a core part of this revolution. It's a force that builds, nurtures, and even tests relationships between brands, influencers, and consumers. As we continue to unpack the various components of this multifaceted dynamic in the upcoming chapters, one thing is certain; social media has a lasting impact on the fitness world. The journey henceforth would explore how one could leverage its features to carve their unique niche in a seemingly saturated market. Like any real journey to fitness, it demands consistency, perseverance, and determination. Buckle up, and let's dive deeper into this fitness realm together!

Chapter 3. Understanding Different Social Media Platforms

Social media has become a cornerstone of modern communication and representation, providing individuals and businesses an avenue for interaction, creativity, and economic opportunity that transcends geographic boundaries. With the advent of various platforms, it can seem daunting to fully explore their intricacies and features, each one catering to different audiences and types of content - text, images, videos, and sometimes a combination of these. In this chapter, we discuss prominent social media platforms, their usage, distinctive features, and audience demographics to guide you in choosing the optimal platform(s) for your fitness brand.

3.1. Facebook: The Social Media Forerunner

Launched in 2004, Facebook is arguably the forerunner of all modern social media platforms that we are familiar with today. With roughly 2.85 billion active users globally, Facebook's expansive user base is diverse in age and location. The largest demographic group are men between the ages of 25 and 34. Facebook Pages, Facebook Groups, and Facebook Marketplace are among its standout features. Fitness business owners can create a page to showcase their services, form groups for customer interaction, and utilize the marketplace for local advertising. Facebook's real-time interaction feature, Facebook Live, provides an avenue to host live workout sessions or Q&As.

3.2. Instagram: The Visual Sweetheart

Acquired by Facebook in 2012, Instagram has emerged as the visual sweetheart of social media. With a primary focus on photo and video sharing, Instagram is often the platform of choice for fitness influencers and brands. Its demographics lean towards a younger audience compared with Facebook, with the majority of its users being under 35. Instagram stories, short-lived posts lasting only 24 hours, and IGTV for longer videos, offer promising ways for fitness brands to share workout routines, in-depth fitness tips, and more. With the Shop feature, businesses can tag products in posts for easy purchase by followers. Fitness brands can capitalize on Instagram's visual nature to share dynamic workouts and before-and-after transformations.

3.3. Twitter: The Real-time Conversation Starter

Twitter, preferred for its brevity and real-time information sharing, stands tall as a platform for rapid-fire communication. Limiting posts or 'Tweets' to 280 characters, the platform appeals to users who want to engage in or follow real-time conversations and debates. Twitter's users are mostly adults aged 18-24, and it has more male than female users. Twitter excels in discussions about real-time events and hence can be utilized by fitness businesses to generate dialogue about ongoing fitness trends, challenges, or industry events.

3.4. YouTube: The Ultimate Video Platform

As a video-sharing platform, YouTube reaches more 18-49-year-olds than any broadcast or cable TV network. It primarily caters to audiences looking for everything from entertainment to educational content. It represents an incredible opportunity for fitness professionals to share in-depth workout routines, nutritional guides, fitness advice, and tutorials with potentially millions of users. Channels can be monetized through ads or channel memberships, offering a return on your content investment.

3.5. LinkedIn: The Professional Hub

LinkedIn is where social media and professional networking converge. At its core, it's designed for career-oriented individuals and business-to-business interactions. Its demographic leans more towards adults aged 25-34. While it may not seem like the traditional go-to platform for fitness businesses, it is particularly suitable for corporate wellness programs or fitness professionals who want to network with others in their industry.

3.6. TikTok: The Rising Star

TikTok, the relative newcomer to the social media landscape and predominantly popular amongst the younger age group (18-24), focuses on short-form, engaging videos under 60 seconds. This platform has amplified trends like snack-sized dance workouts and quick fitness challenges. Fitness brands can leverage the app's viral algorithm to achieve significant reach with fun, engaging videos.

3.7. Snapchat: The Instant Messenger

Although it doesn't have the same broad appeal as more established platforms do, Snapchat's unique offering lies in its time-sensitive content sharing and interactive filters for fun visuals. It's widely popular with younger audiences, particularly those under 24. Fitness brands can take advantage of its features to add an element of fun to their content or to share quick, behind-the-scenes snaps of daily fitness routines.

Navigating social media platforms and their features is an important step towards building your unique fitness brand. By understanding these digital landscapes, you can develop a strategy that resonates with your target audience, encourage engagement, and grow your fitness empire more efficiently and effectively. Remember, the riches are in the niches; understanding which platforms fit your brand best will ensure your time and effort are well invested.

Chapter 4. Building Your Unique Fitness Brand on Social Media

In today's digitally-driven world, carving out a unique brand identity on social media has become crucial for business success, particularly in the fitness industry. Leveraging both the inherent nature of fitness as a visual, engaging activity and the power of social media platforms, it's possible to create an influential fitness brand capable of reaching and impacting millions. This chapter aims to guide you through this process in a detailed and comprehensive manner, covering everything from defining your brand's core values to understanding and connecting with your target audience, to effectively presenting your brand online.

4.1. Define Your Brand

The first step in building a strong brand is definition. Here, you establish the core principles and values of your brand. What makes your workouts unique? How are your health philosophies different from others? Your brand's mission, vision, and values should reflect your unique approach to fitness. Communicate your passion, dedication, and innovation. The more distinct your brand identity is, the more it stands out in the crowded fitness market. Remember, your unique fitness philosophy sets you apart from others, providing something valuable that your audience can connect with.

4.2. Understand Your Audience

Understanding who your target audience is and what they desire is crucial. This knowledge allows you to tailor your branding, content, and messaging to their preferences. Engage with followers, conduct audience research, and pay attention to comments and messages to discover their interests, needs, and fitness goals. By aligning your brand offering with your target audience's needs and aspirations, you can craft a powerful brand narrative that resonates and fosters loyal followers.

4.3. Align Your Brand Across All Social Channels

Each social media platform offers unique opportunities. However, brand consistency across all platforms is crucial. Use the same profile picture, colors, bio, and tone of voice everywhere your brand is represented. This harmonized visual and text presentation bolifies your brand image. For instance, your Instagram page might focus more on visually appealing fitness routines, while your YouTube channel could offer detailed workout tutorials. However, both should unmistakably and articulately communicate your brand's core values and mission.

4.4. Quality Over Quantity

Prioritizing quality content creation is essential. While it's important to post regularly, the quality must not be compromised. High-quality content not only captures the audience's attention but also builds credibility and establishes your brand as a reliable source of information. Offer detailed fitness guides, comprehensive workout videos, informative nutrition tips – all showcasing your unique angle on fitness. Remember, online reputation significantly impacts how your audience perceives your brand. Delaying posting to ensure quality is far better than oversharing mediocre content.

4.5. Engage and Interact

Interactive content is key to building a strong audience connection. Make use of Instagram Stories, Facebook live streams, Twitter chats, or workout challenges to engage your audiences. Offering special incentives, promotions, or contests can also foster stronger community ties and drive user-generated content, providing evidence of your brand's real-world impact. Furthermore, always make sure to respond to comments, messages, and queries promptly and in a genuinely friendly, helpful manner to build a robust online community.

4.6. Leverage Influencer Partnerships

Influencer marketing is a potent tool, particularly in the fitness niche. Collaborating with influencers who align with your brand can expose you to their followers. Make sure the influencers exude the values your brand represents. They should have authentic engagements with their audiences and be seen as trusted sources of fitness advice. Through a well-executed partnership, you can gain credibility, entice new followers, and strengthen your overall brand identity.

4.7. Keep Evolving

Finally, don't be stagnant. As the fitness industry and social media platforms evolve, be willing and ready to innovate and adapt. Use analytic tools to monitor your brand's performance, recognize trends, and gauge audience response. Learn from your mistakes, identify opportunities, and always strive for improvement. This proactive approach will keep your brand relevant, thereby ensuring its longevity.

Building a unique fitness brand on social media is not just about posting workout videos or fitness tips, but about creating a comprehensive, authentic, engaging brand experience. Through commitment, creativity, and strategic planning, you can use the power of social media to position your fitness brand at the forefront of the market, reaching and inspiring individuals worldwide.

Chapter 5. Engaging Your Audience: The Art of Content Creation

Engaging your audience through compelling, timely, and relevant content is an essential aspect of building a robust social media presence. Content creation, in its truest sense, is an art form that involves crafting intricate narratives, forging emotional connections, and inspiring individuals to share your fitness journey and products. As we traverse this integral chapter, you will be introduced to the numerous tactics and strategies on how to captivate your audience and keep them entranced.

5.1. Identifying Your Target Audience

Understanding your audience is the prime step before embarking on the journey of content creation. Various demographic factors such as age, gender, location, and interests should be considered when defining your audience. This segmentation helps tune your content to speak directly to their needs and aspirations. Conduct audience polls, send surveys, invite feedback and study analytics data to create a comprehensive audience persona.

5.2. Crafting a Unique Fitness Narrative

Once you have identified your target audience, narrate a compelling story around your brand marketing. Engage your audience with inspirational fitness journeys, behind-the-scenes glimpses, insightful tips, and transformation stories. A potent narrative resonates with your audience, inspires them to adopt healthier lifestyles, and instills trust in your brand.

5.3. Valuable and Informative Content

One of the key contributors to a successful social media strategy is offering educational and actionable content. This could encapsulate workout routines, diet plans, tips to maintain motivation, lesser-known fitness facts, or even understanding different forms of workout. Providing educational content showcases your knowledge in the fitness space, adds value to the lives of your audience, and keeps them coming back for more.

5.4. Visuals that Speak Volumes

The aesthetic appeal of your content sets you apart from the digital clutter. Opt for clear, high-resolution images, sleek videos, captivating infographics, or engaging GIFs, tailored to the platform you're using. Incorporating professional or homemade graphics can dramatically uplift audience interaction rates.

5.5. Engaging in Real-Time

Building an interactive community plays a vital role in audience engagement. Host live videos, Q&A sessions, IGTV or YouTube webinars, and podcast episodes. This gives your followers a chance to interact with you in real-time and fosters a sense of belonging, thereby enhancing their loyalty to your brand.

5.6. Consistency is Key

Maintaining a regular posting schedule retains your audience's attention and anticipates your posts. Draw up a social media calendar to streamline your content strategy and offer diverse content formats throughout the week.

5.7. Harnessing User-Generated Content

Facilitate your audience to share their fitness journeys, testimonials, and reviews, creating a buzz around your brand. User-generated content (UGC) authenticates your brand, increases audience engagement, and amplifies your reach.

5.8. Experimenting with Content Formats

Experiment with varying content formats - videos, images, GIFs, reels, stories, blogs, podcasts, infographics - to deliver fresh and interesting content. Diversifying your content portfolio reduces monotony and keeps your audience engaged.

5.9. SEO-Optimized Content

Use Search Engine Optimization techniques like keywords, hashtags, and meta descriptions to ensure that your content reaches the right audience. You can also collaborate with other fitness influencers for guest posts or joint workout sessions, optimizing their followers' attention.

5.10. Measuring Success with Analytics

Use analytics tools to track audience engagement, reach, shares, likes, and comments. These metrics help identify what content resonates with your audience and aids in refining your social media strategy.

In conclusion, mastering the art of content creation is a continual process. Continuously innovating, testing, and refining your approach based on audience needs and industry trends is key to sustaining your digital fitness empire. From building an authentic narrative, offering valuable content, creating engaging visuals to harnessing UGC and experimenting with various content formats, every strategy adds a brick to your fitness empire. Stay tuned, consistent, and most importantly, authentic, because, in the digital fitness world, "It's not just about working out, it's about working in!"

Chapter 6. Amplifying Your Reach: Social Media Marketing Strategies

Harnessing the power of the vast social media terrain isn't as effortless as it may seem. It takes strategic planning, meticulous execution, targeted communication, and consistent engagement - a tall order indeed, but immensely rewarding when done right. Let's delve deeper into understanding the ways you can amplify your online presence and reach via effective social media marketing strategies.

6.1. The Power of a Comprehensive Social Media Strategy

A well-structured social media strategy is the North Star guiding your fitness empire's online presence. Without it, you're simply shooting in the dark, hoping for a hit. A comprehensive social media strategy includes identifying your target audience, understanding the type of content they consume, defining your brand's unique selling proposition (USP), and establishing your online brand personality. Conducting regular social media audits and fine-tuning your strategy based on data is equally crucial in this journey.

When building your strategy, don't shy away from extensively studying your competitors, understanding what works for them and what doesn't. This dissection can offer helpful insights into your target fitness community and help mold the backbone of your online strategy.

6.2. Content is King, and Consistency is Queen

The adage "Content is King" holds true even in the realm of social media fitness empires. Without creative, engaging, and timely content, your efforts may turn futile. Your content should be tailored to your fitness audience and be powerful enough to spark conversations, engagements, and shares. High-quality images and catchy captions often do wonders in attracting eyeballs.

On the other hand, the queen - "consistency" - governs how frequently you share your content. Regular posts help keep your brand at the top of your follower's feeds and ensures a steady stream of engagement, thereby increasing your visible footprint.

6.3. Mastering the Art of Engagement

The essence of social media lies in its name - "social." The more you interact and engage with your audience, the more they feel connected to you. Responding to comments, addressing concerns, hosting live chats, and even a mere acknowledgment of a follower's post can significantly boost your engagement rates.

Hosting themed challenges, creating unique hashtags, and regularly seeking follower inputs on various topics helps foster a sense of community, increasing not just engagement but loyalty towards your fitness brand too.

6.4. Optimizing For Platform-Specific Features

Each social media platform offers unique features that can be leveraged for your fitness empire. Instagram's IGTV and Stories, Facebook's Groups and Events, Twitter's Fleets, and Linkedin's Articles - all these features can be exploited to your benefit, allowing you to present a more versatile and dynamic brand image.

For instance, you can use Instagram Stories to share behind-the-scenes footage, host live workout sessions, or present quick fitness tips. Facebook Groups can be utilized to create a community of fitness enthusiasts who can interact, share their progress, and motivate each other.

6.5. Leveraging Social Media Advertising

Platform-specific advertising is an excellent way to boost your reach beyond your organic followers. Through carefully targeted ads, your fitness content can reach those who are most likely to respond to it. Facebook Ads Manager or Instagram Promotions are tools that help you specify audience demographics, interests, and behaviors, ensuring your content gets in front of the right people.

6.6. Influencer Marketing and Partnerships

In the world of fitness, influencers, with their dedicated following, can be your strongest allies. A recommendation from a credible influencer goes a long way in driving traffic to your platform, enhancing brand visibility, and boosting credibility. On the other hand, partnerships with other likeminded fitness brands can result in cross-promotion, widening your platform's reach significantly.

While mastering the social media game may seem daunting, it can be your most powerful tool in building an unforgettable fitness brand. As this journey evolves, you're sure to face challenges, but remember, flexibility and adaptability are keys to thriving in the ever-changing digital landscape. Keep learning, keep trying new things, and most importantly, keep engaging with your community.

Chapter 7. Navigating the Challenges: A Guide to Handling Criticism and Trolls

It is common knowledge that the path to social media success is not always a smooth one. This is particularly true when you are building a fitness brand. Overcoming hurdles such as criticism and dealing with online trolls can be overwhelming. However, understanding their motives, responses, and strategies can significantly minimize their effect on your brand's online reputation.

7.1. Recognizing Motives of Trolls and Critics

Understanding the motives behind criticism can be instrumental in formulating an effective response strategy. Essentially, it is important to distinguish between trolls – users who provoke or harass purely for disruption's sake – and genuine critics who voice their opinions based on actual experience or concern. While the former can be damaging for your brand, the latter can provide valuable insights and areas of growth if handled correctly.

Trolls are often motivated by a desire for attention, a compulsion to cause disruption, or simply out of boredom. They may employ tactics such as; inflammatory comments, provocative posts, or personally attacking other members, all with the goal of causing chaos and drawing attention to themselves.

Critics, on the other hand, may have had a bad experience with your brand, have a better suggestion, or genuinely care about the issue on which they are commenting. Their criticism, while sometimes harsh, is mostly solution-oriented and can provide valuable insights to help your brand improve.

7.2. Dealing with Trolls: Neutralization Strategies

Dealing with trolls is a balancing act, as engaging with them may sometimes only fuel their negative behaviors. However, simply ignoring them can sometimes lead to an escalation of their disruptive activities.

A proactive approach is to create a strong and clear social media policy that defines the line between constructive criticism and trolling. This policy should be visible to all your followers and strictly enforced. Having clear repercussions for crossing the line ensures that your digital platform remains a safe space for positive interaction and healthy discussion.

You can also employ moderation tools available on various social media platforms to help filter out troll activities. Allowing your genuine followers and clients to voice their concerns without being overshadowed or discouraged by the trolls is paramount for customer satisfaction and growth.

7.3. Constructively Responding to Genuine Criticism

It's crucial to understand that no brand is immune to criticism. It's a part of every business trajectory, especially when it involves public engagement on a vast platform like social media. How you respond to such criticisms can have a profound impact on your brand's perception and future growth.

When confronted with genuine criticism, the first step to take is not to react emotionally or defensively. Instead, take time to understand the criticism's root cause and consider it as an opportunity to learn and improve.

A thoughtful, respectful, and transparent response is often appreciated by your audience. They value an entity that is not afraid to admit mistakes and is committed to improving its services or products.

Listening, acting upon the feedback, and showcasing your improvements can turn critics into advocates, and your brand weaknesses into strengths.

7.4. Real-life Scenario: From Critics to Advocates

Let's delve into a hypothetical scenario to better understand this. Suppose you run a fitness brand that promotes protein shakes, and lately, you have received criticism about the high sugar content in your products.

Instead of dismissing these as negative comments, you could respond along the lines of, "Thank you for sharing your concerns about our product's sugar content. We value your feedback and are committed to health and fitness. We are currently reviewing the formulation of our protein shakes, and we assure you that we will take your feedback into account. Please stay tuned for our updates."

This approach assures your critics that their concerns are taken seriously and that your brand is committed to continuous improvement. Following up your words with action will certainly convert some critics into loyal customers and strong advocates for your brand.

7.5. Final Thoughts: Embracing the Challenge

Building and sustaining a fitness brand in the social media age is no small feat. Criticism and trolls are aspects of this digital journey that you cannot wish away. Yet, by acknowledging criticism and tactfully handling trolls, you can steer your fitness brand in the right direction.

Remember to interpret genuine criticism as valuable, actionable feedback. Embrace it as an invitation to improve your services. Keep your social media platforms safe and inviting by managing trolls effectively and promoting an environment of healthy discussions.

Coping with digital criticism and trolls is not just about damage control, but also about growth, evolution, and the continual shaping of your fitness brand. Embrace these aspects as an integral part of your social media journey and make them work for your fitness brand's success.

Chapter 8. Investing in Influencers: Harnessing the Power of Fitness Ambassadors

The power of influencers in broadening the reach of your fitness brand is undeniable. Their popularity, authenticity, and connection with their followers is a potential goldmine for businesses looking to establish a strong brand presence on social media. But what does 'investing in influencers' really entail? How do you harness this power into tangible, business bolstering results? This is what we delve into in this insightful part of our special report.

8.1. The Rise of Fitness Influencers

In the past decade, we have seen a burgeoning growth in the number of Fitness Influencers. These are individuals who have carved out a niche for themselves in the fitness industry through their personalized workouts, nuanced health advice, and unique fitness journey. They share their expertise and fitness lifestyle through captivating content, amassing thousands, if not millions, of loyal followers. This rise can be attributed to the pervasive human tendency to seek inspiration and aspire towards personal growth. In a world increasingly obsessed with health and fitness, fitness influencers have become the new age role models.

8.2. Why Invest in Fitness Influencers?

Investing in fitness influencers can translate into multiple benefits for your brand. Here are a few compelling reasons:

1. Increased Brand Visibility: Leverage the large follower base of influencers to increase your brand visibility across various social media channels.

2. Enhanced Brand Trust: When a well-respected fitness influencer endorses your product or service, it heightens brand trust among their followers.

3. Improved Content Quality: Often, Influencers create high-quality, creative content that can drive engagement.

4. Boost in Sales: Influential endorsements can lead to increases in product sales and subscription sign-ups.

8.3. Identifying The Right Influencer

The secret to a successful partnership often lies in identifying the right influencer in alignment with your brand ethos. An authentic influencer, who shares the same values as your brand and resonates with your target audience, can heighten the impact of your social media campaigns manifold. Here are a few pointers to guide your search:

1. Understand their Audience: Study the influencer's follower demographics to ensure that it aligns with your target market.

2. Analyze their Content: The type, tone, and delivery of their content should harmonize with your brand's image.

3. Track the Engagement Rates: Engagement metrics like likes, shares, comments and saves, gives an indication of their follower's involvement and interaction.

4. Ascertain Authenticity: Gauge the authenticity of the influencers by studying their past collaborations and the transparency in their content.

8.4. Cultivating a Mutually Beneficial Relationship

Investing in influencers goes beyond monetary transactions. It's about building, nurturing, and maintaining a symbiotic relationship with them. Include them in your planning and strategy discussions, respect their creative freedom and offer them growth and learning opportunities. A satisfied and invested influencer can be a long-term asset for your brand, providing continual brand promotion and advocacy.

8.5. Measuring the Impact of Your Influencer Strategy

Finally, it's crucial to evaluate the impact of your influencer marketing strategy. From tracking direct sales and increased website traffic to monitoring brand sentiment and engagement rates, a comprehensive analytical approach will enable you to gauge the effectiveness of influencer marketing for your brand and help tweak your strategy for optimum results.

In essence, investing in fitness influencers is a calculated, strategic maneuver that can provide multiple paybacks for your brand. It is a prominent part of the marketing mix, redefining the way fitness empires are built in the digital world. Harness this power wisely and see your fitness empire flourish. Remember, each influencer collaboration is unique and so will be your journey. Be patient, observant, and ready to adapt as you navigate this new terrain.

Chapter 9. Diving into Data: Utilizing Analytics to Drive Growth

The significance of data in any business venture, particularly in the digital realm, could not be overstated. Today, we begin our excursion through the vast and complex terrain of data analytics, focusing on how it can drive growth in the fitness industry through social media. Presented are an in-depth analysis and procedural steps, from understanding the fundamentals to the application of sophisticated tools and practices to be employed.

9.1. Understanding Analytics and Its Importance

The backbone of this chapter lies in unravelling the crux of analytics first. In simple terms, analytics involves the systematic computational analysis of data which provides valuable insights into user behavior, preferences, and patterns. It's these insights that aid in refining and improving upon your social media strategy to meet the ever-evolving needs of your audience. Imagine having a crystal ball that, instead of glimpsing into the future, reveals a detailed blueprint of your audience's likes, dislikes, engagement time, demographic information, and much more. Wouldn't that be a powerful tool to guide your fitness empire's growth? That's essentially what analytics does.

9.2. The Big Three: Vanity Metrics vs Engagement Metrics vs Conversion Metrics

Next, let's shed light on the three essential categories of metrics found in social media analytics: Vanity Metrics; Engagement Metrics; and Conversion Metrics - each with its distinct value and application.

Vanity metrics, as the name suggests, are head-turning figures that may appear impressive but often don't translate directly into business growth. They include items like the number of followers, page views, and likes. While these metrics are beneficial in understanding the initial reach and visibility, they don't necessarily reflect audience engagement or action.

Engagement Metrics provide a deeper insight into how your followers interact with your content. Shares, comments, average time spent on your page, click-through rates are all part of this category. These metrics reveal how your content resonates with your audience, the kind of content they prefer, the time they are most active, among other things.

Conversion Metrics, the most substantial of the trio, are concrete proof of your social media success - the actual sales, app downloads, newsletter subscriptions, membership sign-ups, or any other action that aligns with your brand's goals.

9.3. Gearing Up: Tools for Social Media Analytics

Typically, each social media platform offers its built-in analytics tool. Facebook has 'Facebook Insights,' Instagram provides 'Instagram Insights,' Twitter supplies 'Twitter Analytics,' and YouTube gives

'YouTube Analytics.' These tools offer a plethora of information, from audience demographics to post-performance.

Apart from these, numerous third-party tools such as Google Analytics, Hootsuite, Buffer, and Sprout Social offer broader, more comprehensive insights. They allow you to measure your performance across multiple social media platforms, track your social media traffic, measure ROI, and even schedule your posts.

9.4. Putting Data into Action: Strategy Building

Having understood the significance of analytics and familiarized ourselves with essential tools, the next leg of the journey is forming strategies based on these insights for growth.

The first port of call is to understand your audience deeply. With demographic data from your analytics, you can come up with content that caters directly to the type of audience you have. Age, gender, location, and active hours each present a valuable piece of the puzzle.

Next, scrutinize your engagement metrics. What type of content receives the most shares? What time do the majority of your audience engage? These insights help you plan your content creation and schedule posts more effectively.

Finally, keep a keen eye on your conversion metrics. Identify which content or campaigns have led to conversions. This analysis can help you design future campaigns that are more likely to hit the mark.

9.5. Stories from the Trenches: Real-World Examples of Successful Use of Analytics

Our journey through the realms of data wouldn't be complete without examining some real-world examples of how fitness empires have leveraged analytics for growth.

For instance, global fitness brand Gymshark's illuminating use of social-media analytics is a lesson in growth. The brand scrutinized its demographic data and found that a significant number of their followers were college students. As a result, they tailored their content and marketing campaigns to appeal directly to this audience – boosting engagement and conversions significantly.

Another example is Nike, with its Nike Training Club app. They used analytics to continuously improve user experience by understanding how users interact with their app. This data-driven approach helped Nike maintain its reputation as a market leader in virtual fitness.

9.6. Taking the Plunge: Practical Tips for Data Analytics

As we round up this meticulous exploration of data analytics, here are some practical tips:

1. Begin with clear, measurable goals.

2. Understand the metrics that matter to your brand.

3. Constantly track and analyze your results.

4. Test different strategies and compare their results.

5. Keep up-to-date with analytics tools and trends.

Data analytics can seem daunting, but its potential is immense. By harnessing its power, you turn raw data into actionable insights, paving the way for your fitness empire's growth in the digital landscape. Take the plunge, dive into the data, and watch your fitness venture thrive.

Chapter 10. Stories of Success: Case Studies from Fitness Social Media Empires

When we speak of success stories, few narrate tales more compelling, inspiring, and profound than the meteoric rise of fitness influencers on social media platforms. Truly, these are the modern-day demigods of fitness and entrepreneurship whose journeys offer us knowledge, inspiration and motivation. So, let's dive in and explore their unique journeys to success.

10.1. The Journey of Kayla Itsines

Kayla Itsines, an Australian personal trainer, author, and entrepreneur, co-founded the fitness empire known as the Bikini Body Guide (BBG). Her journey began in 2008 when she started as a personal trainer at a women's gym in Adelaide. Discovering a universal disdain among her clients for the bulky and masculine physique often associated with conventional fitness routines, she developed a distinctive high-intensity workout regimen. It was designed to promote a lean and feminine 'bikini body', a concept that quickly caught on.

In 2012, she joined Instagram and began posting before–and–after photographs of her clients who had followed her fitness program. The dramatic transformations showcased in these pictorial testimonials resonated with women all over the world, and her Instagram account quickly gained followers by the thousands. Together with her partner Tobi Pearce, Itsines capitalized on this global interest by launching the now-famous Bikini Body Guide in 2014, a series of eBooks accessible to anyone with internet access.

Today, Itsines's BBG program has morphed into an app called Sweat, which offers even more workout and meal plans. Itsines has amassed 12.7 million followers on Instagram and continues to inspire and guide legions of fitness enthusiasts worldwide.

10.2. The Meteoric Rise of Simeon Panda

Simeon Panda, once a regular guy with a passion for fitness, is now revered as one of the world's most influential fitness professionals. From a young age, Panda respected the discipline and dedication it required to keep his body in its best form. His primary goal was never fame rather, he aimed to push his body to its limits and explore his full potential.

When Panda decided to share his fitness journey on social media platforms like Facebook and Instagram, his dedication resonated with millions around the globe. Differentiating himself through a commitment to natural bodybuilding and a relatable, personable nature, he quickly gained a following that multiplied exponentially. His contagious enthusiasm for fitness and a rigorous physical regimen led to a meteoric rise in his influence.

Panda capitalized on his online visibility to launch an array of successful enterprises. These ventures include fitness apparel, nutritional supplements, and an online fitness and diet guide descriptively called 'Mass Gain Extreme.' Panda's journey demonstrates the effective use of personal enthusiasm, a committed fitness regimen, and a clear message to build a successful fitness brand on social media.

10.3. Michelle Lewin: The Face of Fitness

From immigrating to the United States and working in a local car shop, Michelle Lewin's story is about how determination and resilience can lead to worldwide fame in the fitness industry. The Venezuela-born fitness enthusiast transformed her deep passion for fitness into a flourishing career leveraging the power of social media.

She started sharing her fitness journey on social media platforms, notably Instagram, to a rapidly expanding international audience. Her authenticity mixed with her inspiring body transformation fitness routine quickly made Lewin a phenomenon. Today, she is known as one of the most recognizable fitness influencers globally, with a whopping 13.8 million followers on Instagram.

Capitalizing on her success, she has launched fitness products lines and multiple smartphone applications, including "Fitplan," a personal training app providing workouts and fitness plans from professional trainers. Her undeniable impact on the fitness world is a testament to the power of social media.

These engaging narratives featuring Kayla Itsines, Simeon Panda, and Michelle Lewin underpin the undeniable impact of social media on the fitness industry. The commonality amongst their stories lies within their passion for fitness, the empowerment of their followers, being genuine in their approach, and maximizing the opportunities provided by the evolving digital platform. Their stories tell us that with the right approach and sincere dedication, social media can truly take your brand to global heights, building a fitness empire that inspires millions.

Chapter 11. Future Trends: The Next Frontier in Social Media and Fitness

The digital revolution hath transformed the fitness industry beyond measure, ushering in an era where everyone with a smartphone and internet connection has access to a global fitness community. This paradigm shift has seen the rapid growth of fitness empires on social media platforms, leveling the playing field for newcomers while challenging legacy establishments to adapt or perish. As we delve into future trends, it becomes clear that this metamorphosis is only the beginning. The confluence of social media and fitness holds manifold opportunities dominated by technological advancements, new business models, and shifts in consumer behavior.

11.1. Emergence of Gamification in Fitness

In the realm of digital fitness, gamification has emerged as a future trend, creating immersive experiences that cloak the essence of fitness training within compelling, interactive storylines. Fitness apps like Zwift and Peloton have championed this movement, marrying the heart-pounding thrill of video games with gruelling workouts. Users can compete in virtual races, join group workouts, or embark on solo fitness adventures, turning an otherwise monotonous routine into an exhilarating journey.

11.2. Rise of AR and VR in Fitness Workouts

The lines between the physical and digital world are continually blurring with the rise of augmented reality (AR) and virtual reality (VR). Fitness enthusiasts can now perform yoga on a serene beach, lift weights in a high-tech gym, or cycle through picturesque landscapes, all from the comfort of their home. The 'Mirror' workout and 'Oculus Quest's Supernatural' are prime examples of this convergence, transforming the way fitness routines are experienced, making them more engaging, personalized, and immersive.

11.3. Evolution of Micro-influencers in the Fitness Domain

We are witnessing a shift from mega-influencers to micro-influencers in the fitness domain. Micro-influencers, with their modest yet highly engaged follower base, foster a strong sense of community. Their followers often perceive them as trustworthy peers, leading to higher engagement and conversion rates. This shift represents a meaningful opportunity for fitness brands to reach targeted niches more effectively and authentically.

11.4. Increased Emphasis on Mental Health

The growing realization of mental health's paramount importance is shaping the industry. More fitness influencers and brands are promoting from within activities and content centered around mindfulness, stress management, and mental wellness. Expect to see an increase in the blend of mind-body workouts, meditation and mindfulness apps, and content focusing on mental health awareness.

11.5. Adoption of AI-driven Fitness Coaching

AI-driven fitness coaching signifies the growing influence of artificial intelligence (AI) and machine learning (ML). Leveraging these technologies allows for personalized workout plans, nutritional advice, and real-time form corrections, providing users with a holistic, personalized approach to fitness. Companies like Freeletics and Vi embody this trend, offering algorithmically tailored routines that adapt to users' changing performance and goals.

11.6. Surge in Data-driven Personalization

Data-driven personalization will reach new heights in the fitness industry. Fitness trackers and apps can collect real-time data about a person's health and fitness levels, allowing for hyper-personalized workouts and nutrition plans. This personalization extends to social media, where algorithms can deliver tailored fitness content based on user preferences. Expect to see a surge in offerings targeting niche populations, from prenatal workouts to programs designed for older adults.

In conclusion, the boundless potential of the symbiosis between the fitness industry and social media promises an era of innovation and growth. Fueled by pioneering technology and a deep understanding of evolving consumer needs, the intersection of fitness and social media shows no sign of slowing down. Fitness enthusiasts can look forward to an exciting future with more personalized experiences, engaging content, and vibrant online communities. On the other hand, fitness entrepreneurs have an unprecedented opportunity to tap into these emerging trends, adapting their business approaches to harness the promising growth trajectory of the fitness industry's digital frontier.